LUNGS CANCER:

SYMPTOMS, STAGES, AND TREATMENT

By

Daniel Goodweather

TABLE OF CONTENT

INTRODUTION

Disease is a sickness where cells in the body outgrow control. At the point when malignant growth begins in the lungs, it is called cellular breakdown in the lungs.

Cellular breakdown in the lungs starts in the lungs and may spread to lymph hubs or different organs in the body, like the mind. Malignant growth from different organs additionally may spread to the lungs. At the point when disease cells spread starting with one organ then onto the next, they are called metastases.

Cellular breakdowns in the lungs generally are assembled into two primary sorts called little cell and non-little cell (counting adenocarcinoma and squamous cell carcinoma). These kinds of cellular breakdown in the lungs develop contrastingly and are dealt with in an unexpected way. Non-little cell cellular breakdown in the lungs is more normal than little cell cellular breakdown in the lungs.

There are typically no signs or side effects in the beginning phases of cellular breakdown in the lungs, yet many individuals with the condition at last foster side effects including:

a relentless hack

hacking up blood

steady shortness of breath

unexplained sleepiness and weight reduction

a throb or agony while breathing or hacking

You ought to see a GP in the event that you have these side effects.

The significant strategy for anticipation is the aversion of hazard factors, including smoking and air pollution.[14] Therapy and long haul results rely upon the kind of disease, the stage (level of spread), and the individual's in general health.[12] Most cases are not curable.[2] Normal medicines incorporate a medical procedure, chemotherapy, and radiotherapy.[12] NSCLC is some of the time treated with a medical procedure, while SCLC typically answers better to chemotherapy and radiotherapy.[15]

Overall in 2020, cellular breakdown in the lungs happened in 2.2 million individuals and brought about 1.8 million deaths.[5] It is the most normal reason for malignant growth related passing in the two men and women.[16][17] The typical age at finding is 71 years.[1] In many nations the five-year endurance rate is around 10 to 20%,[5] despite the fact that results commonly are more terrible in the creating scene

CHAPTER 1

UNDERSTANDING WHAT LUNG CANCER IS?

After breast cancer in females and prostate cancer in males, the incidence of lung cancer is the third most prevalent major cancer in the United States. Even though lung cancer is still difficult to treat, medical professionals and researchers are making significant progress in detecting it at an earlier stage.

Cancer is a condition in which cells in the body develop in an uncontrolled manner, leading to the disease's name. Lung cancer is the name given to cancer that first develops in the lungs.

The lungs are the initial site of progression for lung cancer, which may then migrate to the lymph nodes or other organs in the body, including the brain. Cancer can spread to the lungs from other organs in the body. The metastases that result from cancer cells spreading from one organ to another are known as metastases.

Small cell and non-small cell lung cancers are the two primary categories that are used to classify the disease (including adenocarcinoma and squamous cell carcinoma). These subtypes of lung cancer develop in distinct ways and respond to treatment in distinctive ways. Cancer of non-small lung cells is far more prevalent than cancer of tiny lung cells. Visit the website of the National Cancer Institute for additional details.

STRUCTURE AND PERFORMANCE OF THE LUNGS IN A NORMAL STATE

The lungs are two organs in your chest that are similar to sponges. The lobes of your right lung can be broken down into three pieces. Your left lung is divided into two lobes. Because the heart takes up more space on the left side of the body, the left lung is smaller than the right lung.

When you take a breath in, air can enter your body through either your mouth or your nose. From there, it travels down your trachea and into your lungs (windpipe). The trachea branches off into smaller tubes that are known as bronchi, which then enter the lungs and continue to branch off into even smaller bronchi. These differentiate into smaller branches that are referred to as bronchioles. Alveoli are the little air sacs that can be found at the terminal end of bronchioles.

When you breathe in air, oxygen is absorbed into your bloodstream, and when you exhale, carbon dioxide is removed from your bloodstream by the alveoli. The primary jobs of your lungs are to take in oxygen and expel carbon dioxide from your blood and body.

The cells that line the bronchi and other sections of the lung, such as the bronchioles and alveoli, are often where lung malignancies begin to develop.

The lungs are encased in a relatively thin layer of tissue known as the pleura. During the process of breathing, your lungs expand and contract, which causes them to slide back and forth against the chest wall. The pleura protects your lungs and facilitates this movement.

Different kinds of lung cancer

There are primarily two different kinds of lung cancer. non-small cell lung cancer (NSCLC). small cell lung cancer (SCLC)

NON-SMALL CELL LUNG CANCER

The most prevalent kind of lung cancer is known as lung cancer with non-small cell differentiation. When you have this condition, cancerous cells begin to form in the tissues of your lungs. Although the progression of non-small cell lung cancer is slower than that of small cell lung cancer, the disease has frequently metastasized by the time it is detected in other parts of the body. Therefore, identification and therapy at an early stage are crucial.

Cancer of the non-small cells of the lung, often known as NSCLC, develops when abnormal cells in the lung tissues proliferate and grow.

What subtypes of non-small cell lung cancer are there to choose from?

Three primary forms of lung cancer are not found in tiny cells:

• Adenocarcinoma This particular form of lung cancer develops in cells that produce mucus and possibly other chemicals as well. The areas of your lung that are closest to your chest cavity are typically where it begins. People who smoke cigarettes regularly or who have smoked in the past are more likely to develop lung adenocarcinoma. However, it is also possible for persons who have never smoked to develop the condition. Additionally, in comparison to the risks associated with other forms of lung cancer, it is more likely to manifest in younger patients.

• Squamous cell carcinoma. Squamous cell carcinoma is a type of lung cancer that typically begins in the core region of the lungs and spreads outward from there. Squamous cells are the flat cells that line the interior of your airways. Having a smoking habit in the past is almost always a contributing factor.

• Large cell carcinoma. This form of lung cancer, which is also known as carcinoma in its undifferentiated state, can develop in any part of the lung. It grows and spreads swiftly, making it more difficult to treat than other diseases.

There are a variety of subtypes of non-small cell lung cancer, the most common of which are adenosquamous carcinoma and sarcomatous carcinoma. These subtypes are seen a lot less frequently.

What are the signs and symptoms of lung cancer that do not originate in tiny cells?

Breathlessness and a persistent cough are two of the most typical early indicators of non-small cell lung cancer. Other symptoms may include chest pain and weight loss. Other possible symptoms of non-small cell lung cancer include the following:

- Soreness or discomfort in the chest.

- A hacking cough that either does not improve over time or grows progressively worse.

- Difficulty in breathing.

- Wheezing.

- Expelling blood when you cough.

- Hoarseness.

- A decreased desire to eat.

- A decrease in body weight for no apparent reason.

- Tiredness.

- Difficulty in the ability to swallow.

- Swelling in the cheeks or the veins in the neck may be present.

Lung cancer can exist asymptomatically for a while until it is identified through screening procedures or routine X-rays.

What are the factors that lead to non-small cell lung cancer?

Even though researchers aren't entirely sure what triggers NSCLC, they have isolated a few potential risk factors. For instance, a significant number of patients diagnosed with NSCLC are current smokers or have a smoking history. Asbestos exposure is another factor that can increase your risk of developing non-small cell lung cancer.

• Being exposed to dust made of minerals and metals.

• Radon, which is a radioactive gas that can be found in nature.

• COPD, which stands for chronic obstructive pulmonary illness (COPD).

• Contamination of the air

• Fibrosis of the lungs (pulmonary).

• HIV\AIDS.

• Radiation to the breast or chest area of the patient

Small-Cell Lung Cancer

Cancer of the small cells of the lung is an extremely rare kind of lung cancer that progresses quickly. Anyone can contract it, but those with a lengthy history of smoking tobacco are most likely to be affected. If a disease is discovered in its early stages, medical professionals can save the lives of some patients while also curing others and extending their lifespan. Quitting smoking is the only method to reduce your risk of developing small-cell lung cancer.

Cancer of the small cells of the lung begins when normally healthy cells in the lungs mutate or transform into malignant cells. After that, these cells begin to divide and multiply out of control. After some time, the malignant cells in your lungs will begin to aggregate into lumps known as tumors.

These tumors might release cancer cells into the body, which your blood or lymph could then pick up and spread to other parts. (The fluid known as lymph moves from one part of your body to another on its way to your lymph nodes.)

Lymph nodes are the common secondary site of dissemination for small-cell lung cancer.

• Bones.

• The adrenal glands. • The liver. • The brain. These glands might be found close to your kidneys.

After the cells have dispersed throughout the body, they may give rise to new malignant tumors in the organs and lymph nodes. A secondary symptom of small cell lung cancer is the accumulation of fluid either within the lungs themselves or in the area around them. It does this by forcing air out of your lungs, which might cause them to collapse.

There are 2 distinct types of SCLC.

There are primarily two different kinds:

• Small-cell carcinoma (oat cell cancer) • Combined small-cell carcinoma

Both conditions contain a wide variety of cells, which proliferate and disseminate in distinct ways. They receive their names from the appearance of the cells when viewed via a microscope.

Several major distinctions may be made between small-cell and non-small-cell lung cancers. Small-cell lung cancer:

• Expands and spreads swiftly. • Develops very quickly.

• Responds favorably to both radiation therapy and chemotherapy, which is the administration of drugs to kill cancer cells (using high-dose X-rays or other high-energy rays to kill cancer cells).

• Is frequently associated with a variety of paraneoplastic syndromes, which are groups of symptoms that are brought on by the production of certain compounds by the tumor.

The Reasons Behind Small-Cell Lung Cancer

• The use of tobacco products is the primary contributor to the development of both small-cell and non-small-cell lung cancers. However, there is a stronger correlation between smoking and small-cell lung cancer than there is between smoking and non-small-cell lung cancer.

Even being exposed to secondhand tobacco smoke can increase your risk of developing lung cancer. If you live with a smoker, your risk of developing non-small cell lung cancer increases by around 30%, and your risk of developing small cell lung cancer increases by about 60%. This is in contrast to those individuals who do not come into contact with second-hand smoke.

People who work in uranium mining are at an increased risk of developing any sort of lung cancer, but small-cell lung cancer is the most prevalent. Those uranium miners who smoke have an even higher incidence rate than those who do not. It is true that radon, an inert gas that results from the breakdown of uranium, has been linked to an increased risk of developing small-cell lung cancer.

The chance of developing lung cancer is considerably increased by exposure to asbestos. The danger is increased even greater when asbestos is combined with another risk factor, such as smoking cigarettes.

Signs and Symptoms of Small-Cell Lung Cancer

In most cases, patients with small-cell lung cancer experience symptoms for approximately two to three months before making an appointment with their primary care physician.

The symptoms may be the result of local growth of the tumor (which refers to growth in the lung where it first appeared), spread to surrounding areas, spread to distant areas, paraneoplastic syndromes, or a combination of some or all of these factors.

Coughing up blood, shortness of breath, chest pain that grows worse with deep breathing, and coughing up mucus are some of the symptoms that can be caused by the local growth of the tumor.

The following is a list of symptoms that may appear as a result of cancer spreading to neighboring areas:

• A hoarse voice as a result of pressure being placed on the nerve that supplies the vocal cords.

• A feeling of shortness of breath caused either by the lungs swelling with fluid or by a compression of the nerve that supplies the muscles of the diaphragm. It is also possible to experience stridor, which is a sound that is created when turbulent airflow passes through a portion of the respiratory tract that is restricted. This happens when the trachea (windpipe) or bigger bronchi are compressed (airways of the lung).

• Difficulty swallowing as a result of pressure on the esophagus (the food pipe) • Swelling of the face and hands as a result of pressure on the superior vena cava This is the vein that carries oxygen-depleted blood back to the lower body from the upper body.

The symptoms caused by cancer that has spread to a distant location depend on where it has spread. Here are several examples:

• If the infection has spread to the brain, you may experience a headache, hazy vision, nausea, vomiting, limb weakness, mental problems, and seizures.

• If it spreads to the vertebral column, you may get back pain as a result.

• If cancer spreads to the spinal cord, it could result in paralysis and the inability to control bowel or bladder function.

• If the condition has spread to the bone, you may experience bone discomfort.

• If cancer has spread to the liver, you may experience pain in the upper right quadrant of your abdomen.

The following are some of the symptoms that can be caused by paraneoplastic syndromes: • Nonspecific symptoms can include tiredness, loss of appetite, and either weight increase or weight reduction.

• Extreme muscle weakness • Difficulty maintaining balance or walking • Alterations in mental status • Alterations in skin color, texture, and facial characteristics • Alterations in the physical appearance of the face and neck

CHAPTER 2

CIGARETTES AND THE RISK OF LUNG CANCER

Tobacco use is still widely acknowledged as the primary contributor to lung carcinogenesis and a host of other disease processes. A change in histology has occurred as a result of the refining of tobacco and the introduction of filters over the past fifty years; as a result, adenocarcinoma has emerged as the most common subtype. Along with several other indicators, smoking has emerged as a powerful prognostic and predictive patient characteristic over the past decade. This article provides a concise assessment of the scientific facts about tobacco, as well as the process and molecular pathways that are involved in the development of lung cancer in smokers and people who have never smoked. In addition to this, the evidence from randomized clinical studies about the effects of smoking on lung cancer outcomes is discussed.

It is estimated that one-third of the world's adult population, which amounts to around 1.1 billion people, is a smoker. This means that one in every six people on the planet is a smoker. Even though smoking-related sickness is often regarded as one of the most preventable causes of death, it is believed to be responsible for approximately 5 million deaths annually across the world. In affluent countries, the rates of smoking have either leveled off or fallen, but in developing countries, smoking-related deaths are on the rise, and the individuals with the lowest levels of education are most likely to be affected by them. At first, more men than women smoked cigarettes, but beginning in the 1980s, there has been a steady narrowing of the gender difference until it reached a plateau.

A school-based cross-sectional survey on water pipe-based tobacco smoking (shisha) in Oman was conducted in 2003, and 1,962 students were questioned for the study. Of those pupils, 26.6% had ever smoked, and 9.6% were current smokers. Only 2.6% of people who are currently smoking are women, compared to 15.5% of male smokers. In the United States of America in the year 2009, roughly 20.6% of adults and almost 20% of high school pupils smoked cigarettes. It is estimated that nine percent of them were users of smokeless tobacco. Products such as wet snuff, chewing tobacco, snus (moist powdered tobacco), and dissolvable nicotine products such as strips and sticks are all examples of smokeless tobacco products. The available research, on the other hand, does not lend credence to the idea that the use of these products is less hazardous than smoking. In addition, there is a significant body of research suggesting that these products may play a role in the development of oral and pancreatic cancers, as well as precancerous oral lesions, gingival recession, gingival bone loss around the teeth, tooth discoloration, and nicotine addiction.

Tobacco usage is the cause of roughly one in five deaths that occur in the United States. According to estimates, the percentage of newly diagnosed cases of lung cancer among males (116,470 cases) and females (109,690 cases) was 14% each in 2012. It was projected that 29% of lung cancer cases in males and 26% of lung cancer cases in females would result in death. At least thirty percent of all cancer fatalities are caused by smoking, and eighty-seven percent of lung cancer deaths are caused by smoking.

Cancers of the small cells of the lung known as small-cell lung carcinoma (SCLC) are extremely uncommon in people who have never smoked. Active smoking also raises the risk of a wide variety of other cancers, such as those of the nasal passages, sinuses, oral cavity, upper aerodigestive tract, pancreas, gynecological system, kidney, bladder, stomach, colorectum, and acute myeloid leukemia. In addition, the risk of developing acute myeloid leukemia is also increased. The World Health Organization (WHO) has released criteria to measure smoking. These standards classify persons as smokers, non-smokers, or ever-smokers, and then construct further sub-categories. In addition, the WHO has produced guidelines to measure secondhand smoke exposure.

Passive smoking, also known as environmental tobacco smoke, is categorized as a recognized human carcinogen and is believed to be the cause of approximately 50,000 deaths per year in the United States. Side stream smoke, which comes from the end of a lighted source (cigarette, pipe, or cigar), contains smaller particles that easily make their way into the cells and is rich in carcinogens. Passive smoking is a mixture of main-stream smoke, which is exhaled by a smoker, and side-stream smoke, which comes from the end of a lighted source (cigarette, pipe, or cigar).

Tobacco smokers' respiratory epithelium frequently contains multifocal premalignant lesions that can occur anywhere along the bronchial tree, as evidenced by a vast body of research dating back to the pioneering work of Auerbach and colleagues. This finding is supported by an extensive body of published research. These findings, which have been referred to as the field cancerization effect, suggest the capability of tobacco carcinogens to substantially mutagenize the respiratory epithelium. [Citation needed] When analyzing premalignant and malignant epithelium from patients with squamous cell carcinoma, Washtub, and co-workers found multiple, sequentially occurring allele-specific chromosomal deletions (loss of heterozygosity) in widely dispersed, apparently clonally independent foci. These findings were made early in the multistage pathogenesis of lung squamous cell carcinoma. In both current and previous smokers, the bronchial epithelium has many foci of genetic alterations, similar to what is observed in patients who have lung cancer. It is important to note that these modifications may continue to exist for a significant amount of time after smoking has been stopped. These enduring anomalies act as a driving force that contributes to higher risk in a population that is rising; the United States is home to more than 45 million ex-smokers, and the majority of newly diagnosed cases of lung cancer are now found in ex-smokers.

In addition to premalignant lesions that are detectable by histologic inspection, studies indicate that smoking generates field effect abnormalities even in histologically normal lung epithelium. These abnormalities can be seen in smokers who have never smoked before. Researchers have utilized high-density gene expression arrays to identify genes in human airway epithelial cells that are changed as a result of smoking cigarettes. It is anticipated that the findings gathered from this research will shed light on the lung cancer risk that smokers face, regardless of whether or not they have COPD. Recent research conducted by Spiral and colleagues suggests that gene expression profiles in histologically normal large airway epithelial cells may be able to function as a biomarker for the existence of lung cancer. These data present a compelling argument in favor of the existence of a widespread airway response to tobacco smoke, even though such a response may not be necessarily evident using traditional histologic examinations. Beane and his colleagues recently proposed a clinic genomic model that has a higher prediction accuracy. This is because the airway gene expression profiles provide important information about the potential development of lung cancer that cannot be adequately predicted by clinically defined risk alone.

Changes in gene expression and cellular functions brought on by smoking tobacco are not limited to the pulmonary airway epithelium alone; they have also been reported in the nasal and buccal epithelium, alveolar macrophages, and peripheral blood. This is because smoking tobacco alters the cytokine environment in the lungs. These findings are in agreement with the concepts that have been provided in the past regarding the systemic inflammatory process that is active in patients who have COPD as well as in patients who have lung cancer.

EPITHELIAL-MESENCHYMAL TRANSITION

Initial descriptions of EMT placed the phenomenon within the context of embryonic development. The epithelial-mesenchymal transition (EMT) is a developmental process in which epithelial cells undergo a transition to a highly motile fibroblastic or mesenchymal phenotype. EMT has been linked to a variety of pathological processes, including chronic inflammation, fibrosis, and the progression of cancer, in addition to its role in embryonic development. EMT is a process that is strictly controlled during normal development. In contrast, the formation and evolution of cancer are characterized by an unregulated EMT, which results in certain aspects of the process is amplified while others are sidestepped. It is now understood that EMT can be influenced in cancer by a variety of different routes. The TGF- pathway, the PI3K/Akt pathway, the ROS pathway, the receptor tyrosine kinase/Ras signaling pathway, and the Want pathway are some examples of those that have been implicated. As a result, EMT is effective in the treatment of a range of cancers, including lung cancer.

Recent research has placed more emphasis on the connection between inflammation and EMT progression in the development of lung cancer as well as resistance to treatment. For instance, IL-1 and PGE2 can suppress the production of E-cadherin, which in turn can promote EMT. These inflammatory mediators can increase the expression of zinc-finger E-box–binding transcriptional repressors of E-cadherin, such as Zeb1, Snail, and Slug, which ultimately results in the advancement of EMT. Recent research conducted in the laboratory of Robert Weinberg hints at a clear connection between EMT and the acquisition of epithelial stem cell characteristics. As a result, inflammation may affect the characteristics of stem cells in the lung cancer pathogenesis process via EMT-dependent processes. EMT-induced alterations have been widely linked to the process of epithelial cancer metastasis. However, research conducted by Mani and colleagues suggests that the EMT genetic program may also regulate early events in the process of carcinogenesis. This links the inflammatory pulmonary environment to both the initiation and progression of lung cancer. The possibility that tobacco and tobacco-specific carcinogens are involved, either directly or indirectly, in the promotion of EMT lends these associations an extra level of significance. For instance, Yoshino and colleagues discovered that benzo[a]pyrene promoted EMT-related genes in lung cancer cells. While fibronectin and Twist were enhanced, the expression of E-cadherin was eliminated. In support of these findings and the setting of another tobacco-induced malignancy, Fontenelle and colleagues discovered that the expression of Twist was impacted by smoking status in patients with bladder cancer. This was found to be the case in the context of bladder cancer. It has also been discovered that the tobacco-specific carcinogen known as 4-(n-methyl-n-nitrosamine)-1-(3-pyridyl)-1-butanone (NNK) can promote EMT in human bronchial epithelial cells through inducing E-cadherin transcriptional repressors.

Epithelial abnormalities brought on by smoking can act in two different ways: first, as targets for abnormal inflammatory responses, and second, as initiators of uncontrolled inflammation. The cytokines, chemokines, and growth factors that are secreted by alveolar macrophages, lymphocytes, neutrophils, endothelial cells, and fibroblasts may be the ones responsible for promoting epithelial dysfunction and the spread of cancer. Some of these connections can be demonstrated most convincingly in mouse models that have been subjected to genetic engineering. For instance, Wisler and colleagues employed KrasLA1 mice, which develop lung adenocarcinoma as a result of somatic activation of the KRAS oncogene, to investigate the significance of ligands for the chemokine receptor CXCR2 in the progression of lung cancer. In the premalignant alveolar lesions of KrasLA1 mice, vascular endothelial cells and neutrophils were shown to have high expression levels of CXCR2 ligands and CXCR2. It is important to note that suppression of CXCR2 prevented the progression of early alveolar neoplastic tumors. These data support other recent research which found that the CXCR2 ligand CXCL8 plays an important part in the development of Kris-induced tumors. These findings show another shared mechanism in the etiology of COPD and lung cancer by pointing the finger at CXCL8 as a possible culprit.

A precipitous rise in the number of people dying from lung cancer was caused by the widespread adoption of cigarette smoking as the primary method of tobacco consumption throughout the 20th century. Tobacco usage is responsible for around 85 percent of all cases of lung cancer; non-smokers can also develop lung cancer as a result of being exposed to secondhand smoke. The risk of developing lung cancer is proportional to the amount of tobacco that is smoked, and this risk cannot be reduced by switching to filtered cigarettes or cigarettes with reduced levels of tar or nicotine. Quitting smoking, particularly when done so at an earlier stage in life, lowers the dose-dependent dangers of tobacco on the development of lung cancer. Tobacco use after a cancer diagnosis is associated with an increase in toxicity, an increase in noncancer comorbidity, an increase in second primary malignancies, a loss in quality of life, and a drop in survival rate in people who have cancer. Quitting smoking can improve health outcomes for patients with cancer as well as individuals who do not have cancer; however, oncologists do not always provide help for quitting smoking on a normal basis to their patients. To lessen the negative impacts that smoking has on one's health, concerted efforts need to be made to lessen one's exposure to smoking, improve methods for reliably assessing smoking in clinical settings, and broaden the availability of assistance for quitting smoking. The recent international initiatives to regulate the use of tobacco and increase lung cancer screening hold the potential of lowering the mortality rate from lung cancer in the future.

CHAPTER 3
SYMPTOMS OF LUNG CANCER

The majority of cases of lung cancer do not present any symptoms until the disease has already progressed to other parts of the body; nevertheless, some individuals who have early lung cancer do experience symptoms. If you take yourself to the doctor as soon as you detect any symptoms, your cancer may be diagnosed at an earlier stage, when it is more probable that treatment will be successful.

It is far more likely that something other than lung cancer is the root cause of the majority of these symptoms. However, if you experience any of these issues, you should make an appointment with your primary care physician as soon as possible to have the root cause identified and, if necessary, addressed.

The following are the most typical symptoms of lung cancer: • A cough that either does not improve over time or grows worse

• Coughing up blood or mucus that has a rusty coloration (spit or phlegm)

• Chest pain that is frequently made worse by activities such as coughing, laughing, or taking deep breaths

• Hoarseness • Loss of Appetite • Weight Loss That Isn't Supposed To Be There

• Difficulty breathing • Feeling fatigued or weak • Infections such as bronchitis and pneumonia that do not go better or keep returning

• Recently developed wheezing symptoms

The following symptoms may present themselves if lung cancer has migrated to other areas of the body: • Pain in the bones (like pain in the back or hips)

• Alterations to the nervous system (such as headaches, numbness or weakness in an arm or leg, dizziness, problems with balance, or seizures), which can result from cancer that has progressed to the brain.

• Jaundice, which is characterized by yellowing of the skin and eyes, as a result of cancer that has progressed to the liver

• Enlargement of lymph nodes, which are collections of immune system cells and can be found in areas such as the neck and the area just above the collarbone

Certain types of lung cancer have been linked to the development of syndromes, which are collections of distinct symptoms.

Horner syndrome

Pancoast tumors are a term that is used to refer to cancers that affect the upper portion of the lungs. Non-small cell lung cancer (NSCLC), rather than small cell lung cancer (SCLC), is the most likely diagnosis for these tumors (SCLC).

Horner syndrome is a collection of symptoms that can be caused when particular nerves in the face and eye are affected by Pancoast tumors. These symptoms include the following:

• drooping or weakening of one upper eyelid • a smaller pupil (the dark portion in the center of the eye) in the same eye • little or no perspiration on the same side of the face as the affected eye

Shoulder pain of a severe nature is another symptom that may be caused by Pancoast tumors.

Superior vena cava syndrome

A big vein known as the superior vena cava (SVC) is responsible for transporting blood from the head and arms to the cardiovascular system. It travels close to the lymph nodes and the upper part of the right lung as it traverses the interior of the chest. In this region, tumors have the potential to push on the superior vena cava (SVC), which can result in a pooling of blood in the veins. As a result, edema may occur in the face, neck, arms, and upper chest area (sometimes with a bluish-red skin color). If it affects the brain, it can also produce headaches, dizziness, and a change in the user's state of consciousness. SVC syndrome can develop gradually over time; but, in certain circumstances, it can become life-threatening and needs to be treated as soon as possible.

Syndromes of paraneoplastic transformation

Some forms of lung cancer generate hormone-like chemicals, which then enter the bloodstream and cause difficulties in distant tissues and organs, even though cancer has not yet migrated to those locations. Paraneoplastic syndromes are the names given to these conditions. These disorders may be the earliest signs of lung cancer in some people. Because the symptoms manifest in a variety of organs, other diseases besides lung cancer can at first be considered to be the likely culprit.

Paraneoplastic syndromes are not exclusive to small-cell lung cancer and can occur in patients with other types of lung cancer as well. The following are some examples of common syndromes:

• SIADH, also known as the syndrome of inappropriate anti-diuretic hormone, is a disorder in which the cancer cells produce a hormone called ADH. This hormone causes the kidneys to retain water. This causes a decrease in the amount of salt found in the blood. Fatigue, loss of appetite, muscle weakness or cramping, nausea, vomiting, restlessness, and confusion are some of the symptoms that can be associated with SIADH. Seizures and coma are possible outcomes for severe instances that do not receive treatment.

• Cushing syndrome: This illness is characterized by the production of ACTH by the cancer cells; ACTH is a hormone that stimulates the adrenal glands to produce cortisol. This can result in symptoms such as increased weight, easy bruising, tiredness, drowsiness, and fluid retention. Other symptoms may include bruising more easily. Additionally, increased blood pressure, elevated blood sugar levels, and even diabetes can be brought on by Cushing syndrome.

• Nervous system problems: SCLC can occasionally prompt the immune system of the body to launch an attack against parts of the neurological system, which can result in a variety of complications. One such condition is known as Lambert-Eaton syndrome, which affects the muscles. The muscles that surround the hips can become weak when this syndrome is present. The inability to rise easily from a seated posture is often one of the earliest warning signals. In time, the muscles that surround the shoulder could become less strong. A condition that is not very common is called paraneoplastic cerebellar degeneration. This condition can lead to problems with speech and eating, as well as a loss of balance and unsteadiness in the movement of the arms and legs. SCLC can also cause additional problems with the neurological system, such as a decrease in muscle strength, altered sensations, difficulties with vision, and even alterations in behavior.

• High calcium levels in the blood, also known as hypercalcemia, can lead to symptoms such as frequent urination, thirst, constipation, nausea, vomiting, stomach pain, weakness, exhaustion, dizziness, and confusion.

• Clots in the blood

Again, the likelihood that lung cancer is the root cause of many of these symptoms is quite low. Other diseases and conditions are far more plausible candidates. However, if you experience any of these issues, you should make an appointment with your primary care physician as soon as possible to have the root cause identified and, if necessary, addressed.

CHAPTER 4
PREVENTION OF LUNG CANCER

Cancer prevention refers to the practice of taking measures to reduce one's risk of developing cancer. The incidence of newly diagnosed cases of cancer in a group or population can be reduced if measures are taken to avoid the disease. We can only hope that this will result in a reduction in the number of deaths caused by cancer.

Researchers investigate both risk factors and preventive factors to forestall the development of new malignancies. Cancer risk factors include everything that raises the likelihood of a person having cancer, while cancer protective factors include anything that lowers the likelihood of someone developing cancer.

Certain cancer risk factors can be prevented, but the majority of them cannot. To give one example, smoking and the inheritance of specific genes both contribute to the development of certain types of cancer; however, only smoking may be avoided. It's possible that maintaining a balanced diet and exercise routine will help ward off certain types of cancer. It is possible to minimize your risk of developing cancer by increasing the number of protective factors and decreasing the number of risk factors, but this does not guarantee that you will not develop cancer. No matter how long you've been a smoker, it's never too late to kick the habit. Every year that you go without smoking reduces the likelihood that you may get major diseases like lung cancer.

If you quit smoking for 12 years, your risk of having lung cancer is reduced to more than half of what it would be for someone who smokes. If you've been smoking for 15 years, your risk of developing lung cancer is essentially identical to that of someone who has never smoked.

The Top Ten Ways to Reduce Your Risk of Developing Lung Cancer

1. Quit smoking

Lung cancer was a condition that was diagnosed relatively infrequently at the turn of the 20th century. The substantial growth can be attributed, in large part, to the rising prevalence of smoking among adults in the United States. In point of fact, it is estimated that almost ninety percent of lung cancers diagnosed in today's society may be traced back to smoking or the inhalation of tobacco smoke.

If you are a woman, smoking raises your chance of having lung cancer by 25.7 times, and if you are a man, it raises your risk of developing lung cancer by 25 times.

Giving up smoking is one of the most important things you can do to reduce your risk of developing lung cancer. According to the findings of certain studies, if you stop smoking after 10 years, your chance of developing lung cancer is reduced by 30 to 50 percent compared to that of persons who continue to smoke.

2. Stay away from secondhand smoke.

The smoke that comes from the cigarettes or cigars of other individuals, in addition to the smoke that those people themselves exhale, is referred to as "second-hand smoke."

When you breathe in second-hand smoke, you are exposing yourself to a significant amount of the toxins that are produced by cigarettes. About 70 of the compounds found in secondhand smoke are known to cause cancer, and the smoke itself contains hundreds more chemicals that are dangerous. Even short periods of exposure to secondhand smoke might have negative health effects.

The Centers for Disease Control and Prevention (CDC) estimates that those who do not smoke but are exposed to secondhand smoke are at an increased risk of developing lung cancer. Each year, this risk results in the deaths of more than 7,300 people.

Even if laws have made it more difficult to be exposed to secondhand smoke in public places, it is still crucial to make every effort to prevent breathing in secondhand smoke at home and in the workplace.

3. Have your property tested for radon gas.

Radon is a radioactive gas that is invisible and odorless; nonetheless, it is the second leading cause of lung cancer, right behind smoking; more importantly, it is the primary cause of lung cancer among those who have never smoked.

The decay of uranium found in rocks and soil results in the production of the radioactive gas known as radon. It is possible for it to enter your home through fractures in the flooring, walls, or foundation. It can also seep into the water supply and the air supply. It has the potential to accumulate in your home over time.

According to the Environmental Protection Agency (EPA), it is estimated that around 1 in every 15 residences in the United States has levels of radon that are above the national average.

It is highly recommended that you get a radon test done on your property. You might choose to purchase a home testing kit or hire a specialist in order to have your home checked for the presence of this gas. If you discover excessive levels of radon in your home, a professional can offer recommendations on how to bring those levels down to safe levels.

4. Be familiar with your family's past.

You have up to twice the risk of developing lung cancer compared to persons who do not have a family history of the disease if an immediate family member (such as a parent or sibling, for example) has had lung cancer. This elevated risk is caused by both hereditary and environmental factors working together.

It is imperative that you contact your primary care physician if anyone in your immediate family develops lung cancer, regardless of whether or not they smoked cigarettes. They might suggest various screenings as a way to assist in lowering your risk.

5. Avoid contact with harmful substances

The risk of developing lung cancer is increased when a person is exposed to certain substances. A few examples of them are as follows: asbestos; arsenic; nickel; soot; cadmium; silica; and diesel exhaust.

Your risk will increase in proportion to the extent of your exposure.

Your place of employment is the setting in which you are most likely to come into contact with these toxins. If these compounds are present in your place of employment, you should make every effort to protect yourself by using protective gear and reducing the amount of time you spend exposed to them.

6. Take steps to lower your chance of contracting HIV.

The human immunodeficiency virus, also known as HIV, has been connected to an increased likelihood of developing lung cancer. In point of fact, studies have shown that it may increase your risk of acquiring lung cancer by a factor of two.

There are a number of potential causes for an increased chance of developing lung cancer, some of them are as follows:

- HIV generates a greater level of inflammation throughout the body. • The HIV infection has repercussions. • The smoking rate is higher among people with HIV.

When engaging in sexual activity, it is imperative that you always use a condom in order to lower your chance of contracting HIV. You should also think about getting tested on a frequent basis, especially if you engage in sexual activity without protection or use medicines that are administered intravenously.

7. Protect your chest as much as possible from radiation.

Radiation with a high energy level, such as X-rays, gamma rays, and other forms of radioactive waves, has the potential to cause damage to your DNA and raise your risk of developing cancer.

Certain medical treatments can damage the cells in your lungs, which can increase your risk of developing lung cancer. This comprises diagnostic tests such as a chest X-ray; a CT scan; a pet scan; and so on and so forth.

- radiotherapy and radiation

The likelihood of developing cancer as a result of these treatments is extremely remote, and the potential benefits often outweigh the dangers.

However, you should discuss the possibility of safer alternatives with your physician, particularly if you have additional conditions that increase your risk of developing lung cancer.

8. Get frequent exercise

According to some studies, engaging in regular physical activity can cut the chance of developing lung cancer by as much as 20 to 30 percent in women and by 20 to 50 percent in men. It appears that the more you exercise, the more danger you reduce for yourself.

Exercise may reduce the risk of developing lung cancer by a number of mechanisms, including but not limited to the following: increased lung function; improved immune function; reduced inflammation; lower levels of carcinogens in the lungs; improved ability to repair DNA. However, experts are not entirely clear on the nature of this connection.

The research has not yet provided a definitive answer regarding the exact mechanism through which physical activity reduces risk. This is made more difficult by the fact that smokers typically have lower rates of physical activity than non-smokers do on average.

9. Follow a nutritious eating plan.

In addition, the foods you eat are a significant factor in determining your risk of developing cancer. Consume a diet rich in fruits and vegetables, whole grains, and lean proteins to reduce the likelihood of developing cancer and other diseases.

There are also certain foods that, according to a study, can help prevent lung cancer. Some examples of these meals are cruciferous vegetables such as Brussels sprouts, cabbage, cauliflower, and broccoli.

• turmeric

• Green tea

10. Speak with your primary care physician about getting screened.

Regular screening for lung cancer is something you should consider doing if you have a history of smoking and your age puts you at a higher risk of developing lung cancer. Screening can assist in the early detection of lung cancer, when the disease may be more amenable to treatment.

Screening, on the other hand, is something that is only recommended for persons who have a high risk of developing lung cancer. Talk to your primary care physician if you have any reason to believe that you could qualify for screening and want to find out more information.

CHAPTER 5

RADIATION THERAPY

X-rays are the name given to the high-energy beams that are used in radiation therapy for the treatment of lung cancer. It is particularly effective at controlling or eliminating tumors in specific areas of the body and can improve a patient's prognosis. [Case in point:] [Case in point:]

At the Memorial Sloan Kettering Cancer Center, we use radiation treatment to treat patients whose lung malignancies have been restricted to the chest but cannot be removed surgically. These patients have been diagnosed with stage I or stage II disease. We are now able to deliver potent doses of radiation straight to your tumor with a high degree of accuracy by making use of the most recent and cutting-edge technologies. When compared to more conventional methods, some of the ways that we implement can cut down on the total number of radiation treatments that you have to do while simultaneously lowering the likelihood that you will experience adverse effects.

Different kinds of radiation treatment

Radiotherapy applied to the body in a stereotactic fashion

Stereotactic body radiation therapy, often known as SBRT, targets cancer cells specifically and administers very high doses of radiation to those cells. It requires the utilization of cutting-edge image guidance technology, which can detect the precise position of a tumor in all three dimensions. SBRT makes it possible to administer substantial radiation doses in a relatively limited number of treatment sessions. The term for this method of treatment is called low-fractionated radiation therapy. Our radiation oncologists at MSK use a sort of hypo fractionated radiation therapy called MSK, which is able to give these high doses with a high degree of accuracy. This treatment is typically reserved for the early stages of the disease when the tumor is still relatively small and cancer has not spread beyond the lungs. Our group has a wealth of experience applying this method, and we have been successful in managing tumors 90% of the time with very few adverse effects.

Radiation therapy with intensity-modulated beams

In the fight against lung cancer, our radiation oncologists were among the first to implement intensity-modulated radiation therapy, often known as IMRT. After a CT scan that creates a three-dimensional map of the tumor, with intensity-modulated radiation therapy (IMRT), complex computer systems are used to determine and provide individualized doses of radiation to the tumor from a variety of directions. This makes it possible to provide a high dosage of radiation to lung tumors, particularly those that include the central tissues in the chest such as the lymph nodes. This is particularly useful for treating cancers of the lung that have spread to these structures.

When planning treatment, we make use of both regular CT scans and PET imaging due to the fact that it might be difficult to differentiate tumor cells from normal tissue that is close when utilizing typical CT scans. With the help of PET technology, our doctors are able to more accurately and safely target the tissue that contains cancer cells, allowing them to avoid damaging healthy tissue in the process.

Using IGRT to the chest, we treat roughly 400 patients each year who have non-small cell lung cancer. This treatment is also used for lung cancer that has progressed to other parts of the body.

Therapy using Protons

Our radiation oncologists are able to administer proton treatment for certain instances of lung cancer. Protons, rather than x-rays, are the type of radiation that is used in this cutting-edge form of radiation treatment, which is used to treat tumors that may be tough to eradicate with normal radiation. Our doctors are able to deliver the necessary dose to the tumor, which increases the likelihood that it will be destroyed, while simultaneously lowering the dose that is delivered to normal tissues. This is made possible by proton therapy, which directs the energy that fights cancer to specific locations within the body. At the moment, this cutting-edge technology is only accessible in a select few areas across the United States.

Brachytherapy

There is a possibility that brachytherapy could help certain patients who have lung cancer. In order to reduce the likelihood of cancer coming back after treatment, this technique entails inserting radioactive material that has been hermetically sealed inside a tiny tube into the body during surgery. Endobronchial brachytherapy is a specific method that allows us to send high doses of radiation to the airways. This allows us to treat lung cancer more effectively. There are certain patients who may benefit from this sort of radiation therapy, specifically those whose cancer has spread to the bigger airways.

Clinical Investigations in the Field of Radiation Oncology

The MSK lung cancer team is a world leader in clinical studies that test innovative radiation treatments or radiation therapy combined with surgery and chemotherapy. These trials are conducted at MSK and other leading institutions across the world.

The precision of both our imaging and radiation administration methods is a primary focus of many of the clinical trials that we are now conducting. Our objective is to administer radiation therapy in a way that causes the least amount of harm to the normal tissues adjacent to the tumor while achieving the highest possible degree of success in treating cancer.

In addition, we are conducting research on numerous targeted medications in conjunction with radiation treatment in order to gain a better understanding of the relationship between radiation therapy and the immune system in the battle against cancer.

Gating of the respiratory system

Many tumors, including those that are located close to the lungs, move as a direct result of breathing and other involuntary motions that occur throughout the body. The radiation therapy team is able to "paint" more concentrated doses of radiation onto tumors with higher accuracy thanks to a technique called respiratory gating. During radiation therapy, the device monitors the mobility of the tumor caused by breathing, which enables the medical team to better target the cancerous growth while preventing healthy tissue from being exposed to radiation that is not essential.

Rapid Arc

In order to provide IMRT in a more timely and accurate manner, the care team may make use of the Rapid Arc technology. The duration of treatment can be decreased using a technique called rapid arc radiation therapy. A linear accelerator makes a single complete rotation around the patient, delivering a sculpted and tightly focused beam of radiation directly to a tumor in under two minutes. This process takes place in less than two minutes. This leads to improved targeting of the tumor while causing less damage to the healthy tissue that is surrounding it. Additionally, it assists in shortening the total duration that a patient must undergo radiation treatment.

Radiation's potentially fatal effects on lung cancer patients

Radiation therapy has the potential to create adverse effects, some of which may require additional medical attention. These potential adverse effects may include, but are not limited to inflammation, redness, or blistering of the skin; pain; fatigue; loss of hair in the area where radiation was administered;

When radiation therapy is administered in conjunction with other therapies, such as chemotherapy, the adverse effects could be more severe.

CHAPTER 6

THERAPY FOR PATIENTS WITH LUNG CANCER

The management of treatment for lung cancer is handled by a team of specialists from many departments that collaborate in order to offer patients the most effective treatment available.

This team consists of the medical professionals who are necessary to make a diagnosis, determine the stage of your cancer, and arrange the most effective therapy for you. If you are interested in learning more, speak with either your physician or nurse on this matter.

The treatment that you receive for lung cancer is determined by a number of factors, such as the type of lung cancer that you have (non-small-cell or small-cell mutations on cancer); the size and position of cancer; the stage at which your cancer has progressed; and the size and position of cancer.

- the state of your health in general

It can be challenging to choose which treatment would be most beneficial for you. Your oncology team will provide you with recommendations, but it will be up to you to make the final choice.

Surgical procedures, radiation therapy, chemotherapy, and immunotherapy are the most prevalent forms of available treatment. A mix of these therapies might be recommended for you, depending on the type of cancer you have and the stage it is at.

Your treatment plans

Whether you have non-small-cell lung cancer or small-cell lung cancer will determine the treatment approach that your doctor recommends for you.

Non-small-cell lung cancer

If you have non-small-cell lung cancer that is located in only one of your lungs and you are in generally good condition, the malignant cells will most likely be removed surgically if you have this type of lung cancer.

After this, you might get a round of chemotherapy to eliminate any cancer cells that may still be present in your body after the previous treatment.

You may be offered radiotherapy as a technique of eliminating cancerous cells if cancer has not progressed very far but surgery is not a viable option for you (for instance, due to the fact that the state of your general health places you at an elevated risk of problems). Combining this treatment with chemotherapy is an option in some instances (known as chemoradiotherapy).

Chemotherapy and/or immunotherapy are typically indicated when standard cancer treatments, such as surgery or radiotherapy, are no longer likely to be successful due to cancer's advanced stage.

If, after receiving chemotherapy treatment for your cancer, cancer begins to grow once more, a different treatment plan may be suggested to you.

In certain instances, if cancer has a particular mutation, a biological or targeted therapy may be advised as an alternative to chemotherapy, or after chemotherapy has been completed.

Biological therapies are pharmaceutical treatments that slow down or halt the progression of cancer cells.

Small-cell lung cancer

Chemotherapy is the standard treatment for small-cell lung cancer. This treatment may be administered on its own or in conjunction with radiotherapy or immunotherapy.

This has the potential to both extend people's lives and alleviate their problems.

In most cases, the treatment for this kind of lung cancer does not involve surgery. This is due to the fact that by the time cancer is properly recognized, the disease has typically already progressed to other parts of the body.

On the other hand, surgery is an option for treatment if the cancer is discovered at an extremely early stage. In certain particular instances, chemotherapy or radiotherapy may be used following surgery in order to assist in lowering the likelihood of cancer coming back.

Surgery

There are three primary categories of lung cancer surgery, which are as follows:

• lobectomy, which refers to the removal of one of the lobes, which are the major sections of the lung. If the cancer is contained in just one part of one lung, your doctors may recommend that you have this operation.

• pneumonectomy, which refers to the removal of the complete lung. When the cancer is located in the middle of the lung or when it has spread across the lung, this treatment option is used.

• wedge resection or segmentectomy, in which a segment or wedge-shaped portion of the lung is surgically removed. This technique is only appropriate for a select few people at any one time. You will only be offered this treatment if your physicians believe that the cancer is localized to a single section of your lungs. In most cases, this is a stage of non-small-cell lung cancer that is extremely early on.

If part or all of your lung needs to be removed, you may be anxious about how you will be able to continue breathing, however, it is feasible to maintain regular breathing with one lung.

Having difficulty breathing prior to surgery increases the likelihood that you will continue to struggle with this symptom following the procedure.

Examinations prior to the operation

Before your surgery, you will need to undergo a series of examinations that will evaluate both your overall health and the capacity of your lungs. These may include the following:

• an electrocardiogram (ECG), in which electrodes are placed on your chest in order to monitor the electrical activity of your heart. • a lung function test is known as spirometry, in which you will breathe into a machine in order to determine how much air your lungs are able to breathe in and out. • an exercise test, in which you will run on a treadmill in order to determine your aerobic capacity.

How it is actually done

During surgery, an incision is typically made in the patient's chest or side in order to remove a portion of the diseased lung or the entire lung altogether.

This procedure is known as a thoracotomy.

If it is believed that cancer has progressed to nearby lymph nodes, then those lymph nodes may also need to be removed.

There is also a complementary technique available known as video-assisted thoracoscopic surgery (VATS), which might be appropriate in certain cases. In this form of keyhole surgery, only very small incisions are done in the chest area of the patient.

During the procedure, the surgeon will implant a small camera into one of the incisions so that they can view the interior of your chest on a monitor as they cut out the afflicted portion of your lung.

Following the surgical procedure

Following your procedure, you will most likely be discharged between 5 and 10 days later. On the other hand, getting back to normal after having lung surgery can take several weeks.

After your procedure, you will be given the go-ahead to begin moving around as soon as humanly possible. Even if you are required to remain in bed, you should continue to move your legs on a regular basis in order to improve your circulation and reduce the risk of developing blood clots.

You will be guided through some breathing exercises by a physiotherapist in order to assist prevent difficulties.

When you get back to your house, you'll need to do some light exercise to keep your strength and fitness levels up.

After receiving therapy for lung cancer, recommended kinds of exercise that are appropriate for the majority of patients include walking and swimming.

Have a conversation with your care team about the different sorts of physical activity that are appropriate for you.

Complications

Lung surgery, like any other type of operation, presents the possibility of experiencing problems.

In most cases, they can be treated with medication or more surgery, which may require you to remain hospitalized for a longer period of time.

The following are examples of complications that can arise from lung surgery: inflammation or infection of the lung (pneumonia); excessive bleeding;

• a blood clot in the leg (deep vein thrombosis), which has the potential to go up to the lung and cause serious complications (pulmonary embolism)

Radiotherapy

Radiotherapy involves exposing patients to brief bursts of radiation in order to kill cancer cells. It is possible to treat lung cancer with a variety of different methods with this substance.

If you are not in good enough health to have surgery for non-small-cell lung cancer, an extensive course of radiotherapy, often known as radical radiotherapy, is an option for treating the disease.

It's possible that a specialized form of radiotherapy known as stereotactic radiotherapy could be used instead of surgery to treat very small tumors.

When a cure for cancer cannot be achieved, radiotherapy may be used to manage symptoms such as pain and the production of bloody coughing fits, as well as to slow the progression of the disease (this is known as palliative radiotherapy).

Prophylactic cranial irradiation, often known as PCI, is a form of radiotherapy that is sometimes used in the treatment of small-cell lung cancer.

PCI entails administering a relatively modest dosage of radiation to the patient's entire brain.

Because there is a possibility that small-cell lung cancer can spread to the brain, this is done as a prophylactic precaution.

The mode of administration for radiotherapy

The following are the three primary applications of radiotherapy:

• the more traditional form of radiotherapy, known as external beam radiotherapy, in which beams of radiation are focused on the areas of your body that are afflicted.

• Stereotactic radiotherapy is a more accurate type of external beam radiotherapy in which many high-energy beams deliver a higher dose of radiation to the tumor while avoiding the surrounding healthy tissue as much as possible. This type of radiotherapy was developed in the 1970s.

• insertion of a catheter, which is a very tiny tube, into your lung as part of internal radiation. After traveling via the catheter and being positioned against the tumor for a few minutes, the radioactive material is then withdrawn.

External beam radiotherapy is utilized more frequently than internal radiotherapy for the treatment of lung cancer, particularly if it is believed that a cure may be achievable.

Because stereotactic radiation is more effective than normal radiotherapy alone in the treatment of tumors of this size, it can be utilized to treat cancers that are extremely early in their stages.

When your airway is completely blocked or partially blocked by cancer, a palliative treatment called internal radiation is typically recommended.

Different methods of therapy

The course of radiotherapy treatment can be organized in a variety of distinct ways.

People who undergo conventional radical radiation typically undergo somewhere between 20 and 32 sessions of treatment.

In most cases, patients receiving radical radiotherapy receive treatment five days per week, with the weekends off. Each session of radiation lasts for ten to fifteen minutes, and the entire course of treatment typically lasts between four and seven weeks.

An alternate method of administering radical radiotherapy is known as continuous hyper fractionated accelerated radiotherapy or CHART for short.

The CHART is presented three times each day for a total of twelve consecutive days.

Because of the increased radiation dose that is delivered during each session of stereotactic radiotherapy, the number of treatment sessions required is reduced. Patients undergoing stereotactic radiation often undergo anything from three to ten treatment sessions.

The number of sessions required for palliative radiation typically ranges from one to five.

Concomitant effects

Radiation therapy to the chest may cause a variety of side effects, including • fatigue (tiredness); • a persistent cough that may bring up blood-stained phlegm; • difficulty swallowing (dysphagia); • redness and soreness of the skin, which looks and feels like sunburn; • difficulty breathing (hypoventilation); and • difficulty breathing (hypoxemia).

• a thinning of the hair on your chest

A significant number of persons who undergo radiation report only experiencing moderate side effects or none at all.

However, there is a possibility that you will have some negative effects both during and after therapy.

Talk to your healthcare provider or a nurse if you have any questions regarding the potential for side effects or how to treat them.

In addition, consult a doctor if you are concerned about the symptoms you are experiencing.

Chemotherapy

Chemotherapy is a method of treating cancer that makes use of potent cancer-killing medicines. Chemotherapy is an effective treatment option for lung cancer and can be administered in a number of different methods. For instance, it can be administered: • before surgery to reduce the size of a tumor, which can enhance the likelihood that the surgery will be successful (this is something that is often only done as part of a clinical trial); • after surgery to prevent cancer from coming back; and so on.

When a cure for cancer cannot be achieved, chemotherapy and radiation therapy are combined in order to alleviate cancer's symptoms and halt the disease's progression.

Treatments for chemotherapy are frequently administered in cycles.

A cycle of chemotherapy consists of taking medication for many days straight, followed by a break of several weeks in order to give the treatment time to take effect and for your body to recover from the side effects of the treatment.

The type and stage of lung cancer you have will determine the number of cycles of treatment you require.

The majority of patients require four to six treatment cycles spread out over three to six months.

After the conclusion of these cycles, you are scheduled to visit your physician. It is possible that you will not require any more therapy for cancer if it has improved.

If cancer has not improved after these cycles of chemotherapy, your physician will discuss the possibility of switching to a new kind of treatment. Alternatively, you might need to undergo chemotherapy treatment for maintenance in order to keep cancer under control.

A number of different drugs are typically administered concurrently during chemotherapy treatment for lung cancer.

The medications are typically administered intravenously, which means that they are poured slowly into a vein, or via a tube that is attached to one of the blood vessels in your chest.

Instead of oral medication, certain patients may be given capsules or pills to ingest.

Before beginning chemotherapy, your physician may give you a vitamin injection or write you a prescription for some vitamins to take on your own.

These may help mitigate some of the negative effects of the treatment.

Concomitant effects

Some of the potential negative effects of chemotherapy are as follows: • tiredness

• mouth ulcers • hair loss • a sense of being sick • actual sickness

You may be able to take other medications in addition to your chemotherapy in order to lessen the discomfort caused by these side effects while you are undergoing treatment, or the side effects should progressively go away when treatment is over.

Chemotherapy can reduce the effectiveness of your immune system, leaving you more open to the risk of contracting an infection.

Notify your care team or your primary care physician as soon as possible if you suddenly feel sick or if you have symptoms of an infection, such as a high temperature or other general symptoms of illness.

Immunotherapy

Immunotherapy refers to a range of treatments that work by encouraging the body's immune system to hunt down and destroy cancer cells. It is possible to use it by itself or in conjunction with chemotherapy.

Pembrolizumab and atezolizumab are two examples of immunotherapy drugs that are utilized in the treatment of lung cancer.

It's possible that immunotherapy will be administered to you via a tube made of plastic that is inserted into either a major vein in your chest (a central line) or a vein in your arm (cannula)

The administration of a dose can take anywhere from thirty to sixty minutes, and it is possible that you will need a dose every two to four weeks.

Immunotherapy may be administered for a period of up to two years in patients who experience favorable outcomes and for whom the treatment's adverse effects are manageable.

Immunotherapy frequently causes the following adverse effects: feeling fatigued or weak; experiencing nausea and/or vomiting; feeling ill; having diarrhea; losing your appetite; experiencing pain in your joints or muscles; experiencing shortness of breath.

• alterations in the condition of your skin, such as your skin becoming drier or itchier

Talk to your healthcare provider or a nurse if you have any questions regarding the potential for side effects or how to treat them.

In addition, consult a doctor if you are concerned about the symptoms you are experiencing.

Personalized medicine or targeted medicines

Targeted therapies, sometimes referred to as biological therapies, are prescription medications that have been developed specifically to inhibit the progression of advanced non-small cell lung cancer.

Targeted therapies are only an option for patients if their malignant cells have certain proteins.

In order to determine whether or not these therapies are appropriate for you, your physician may decide to perform a biopsy and run tests on the cells that are extracted from your lung.

The following are some of the adverse reactions that might occur as a result of taking targeted therapies: • flu-like symptoms such as chills, high temperature, and muscle pain • exhaustion • diarrhea • loss of appetite • mouth ulcers • feeling sick to your stomach

Alternative treatments

In addition to surgery, radiation, and chemotherapy, there are a variety of alternative treatments that are occasionally utilized in the management of lung cancer.

Radiofrequency ablation

In the early stages of non-small-cell lung cancer, ablation using radiofrequency may be employed as a treatment option.

A CT scanner is used by the physician as a map to direct a needle to the location of the tumor.

After the needle has been inserted and the tumor has been compressed, radio waves will be transmitted through the needle. The heat that is produced by these waves is what finally puts an end to the cancer cells.

The risk of developing a pocket of air that is stuck between the inner and outer layers of your lung is the most typical risk associated with radiofrequency ablation (pneumothorax).

This condition can be treated by inserting a tube into the lungs in order to expel the air that has become trapped there.

Cryotherapy

Cryotherapy is an option for treatment if cancer progresses to the point where it blocks your airways. This condition, also known as endobronchial blockage, can result in a variety of symptoms, including but not limited to: difficulty breathing a cough coughing up blood

Cryotherapy is carried out in a manner that is analogous to that of internal radiation; however, rather than making use of a radioactive source, a device known as a cryoprobe is brought into contact with the tumor.

The cryoprobe is capable of generating extremely cold temperatures, which assist in the reduction of the size of the tumor.

Treatment with photodynamic light

Photodynamic therapy, also known as PDT, is an alternative treatment option for early-stage lung cancer in patients who are unable or unable to undergo surgery. Additionally, it might be utilized to eliminate a tumor that is obstructing the airways in the body.

Two steps are involved in the process of photodynamic treatment.

To begin, you will receive an injection of a medication that, once it has taken effect, will cause the cells in your body to become hypersensitive to light.

After a delay of between 24 and 72 hours, the subsequent step is performed. A laser is shone through a small tube that is inserted into the body and steered to the location of the tumor.

The laser beam eliminates the malignant cells, which are now more vulnerable to being killed by light than they were before.

Inflammation of the airways and accumulation of fluid in the lungs can both be side effects of photodynamic therapy (PDT). Both of these adverse effects might produce tightness in the chest as well as pain in the lungs and throat. On the other hand, you should begin to feel better as time goes on and your lungs begin to recover from the effects of the medication.